KEEP
CALM

YOU'RE

HAVING A

BABY

KEEP
CALM

YOU'RE

HAVING A

BABY

KEEP
CALM

YOU'RE

HAVING A

BABY

KEEP
CALM

YOU'RE

HAVING A

BABY

KEEP
CALM

YOU'RE

HAVING A

BABY

KEEP
CALM

YOU'RE

HAVING A

BABY

KEEP

KEEP

KEEP

KEEP CALM YOU'RE HAVING A BABY

KEEP CALM YOU'RE HAVING A BABY

KEEP CALM YOU'RE HAVING A BABY

KEEP CALM YOU'RE HAVING A BABY

KEEP CALM YOU'RE HAVING A BABY

KEEP CALM YOU'RE HAVING A BABY

KEEP CALM YOU'RE HAVING A BABY

KEEP CALM YOU'RE HAVING A BABY

KEEP CALM YOU'RE HAVING A BABY

KEEP CALM YOU'RE HAVING A BABY

KEEP CALM YOU'RE HAVING A BABY

KEEP CALM YOU'RE HAVING A BABY

KEEP CALM YOU'RE HAVING A BABY

KEEP CALM YOU'RE HAVING A BABY

KEEP CALM YOU'RE HAVING A BABY

KEEP CALM YOU'RE HAVING A BABY

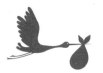

KEEP
CALM
YOU'RE
HAVING A
BABY

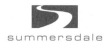

summersdale

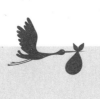

To...

From...

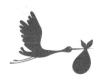

A new baby is like the beginning of all things – wonder, hope, a dream of possibilities.

Eda LeShan

For the hand that
rocks the cradle is
the hand that rules
the world.

William Ross Wallace

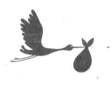

Sometimes… the smallest
things take up the most
room in your heart.

A. A. Milne

The family is one of nature's masterpieces.

George Santayana

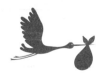

Babies are such
a nice way to
start people.

Don Herold

Being pregnant was
the healthiest I've ever
been in my life. Except
for the cupcakes.

Ashlee Simpson

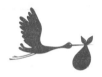

Babies are always more trouble than you thought – and more wonderful.

Charles Osgood

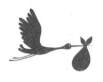

A mother's happiness is
like a beacon, lighting up
the future but reflected also
on the past in the guise of
fond memories.

Honoré de Balzac

The raising of a child
is the building of a
cathedral. You can't
cut corners.

Dave Eggers

Love crawls with the baby, walks with the toddler, runs with the child, then stands aside to let the youth walk into adulthood.

Jo Ann Merrell

I've got my figure back after giving birth. Sad, I'd hoped to get somebody else's.

Caroline Quentin

It is a wise father that
knows his own child.

William Shakespeare

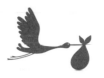

Let us make
pregnancy an
occasion when we
appreciate our
female bodies.

Merete Leonhardt-Lupa

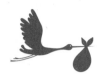

Mother is the name for
God in the lips and hearts
of little children.

William Makepeace Thackeray

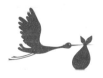

No animal is so
inexhaustible as an
excited infant.

Amy Leslie

We made a wish and
you came true.

Anonymous

When my baby was born…
I suddenly was so full of
love that it was a little bit
as if I was drugged.

Anne-Marie Duff

When you look at
your life the greatest
happinesses are
family happinesses.

Joyce Brothers

A baby is an
inestimable blessing
and bother.

Mark Twain

In every conceivable
manner, the family is link
to our past, bridge to
our future.

Alex Haley

Always end the name of
your child with a vowel,
so that when you yell, the
name will carry.

Bill Cosby

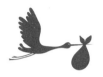

I have a wonderful joy
in a wonderful way
and my wonderful joy
has come to stay.

Florence Scovel Shinn

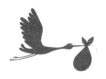

Govern a family
as you would
cook a small fish
– very gently.

Chinese proverb

Parenthood is a lot
easier to get into than
out of.

Bruce Lansky

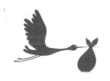

A person's a person,
no matter how small!

Dr Seuss

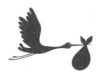

I'd like to be the ideal
mother, but I'm too busy
raising my kids.

Anonymous

Rejoice with your
family in the beautiful
land of life.

Albert Einstein

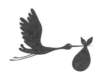

People who say they
sleep like a baby usually
don't have one.

Leo Burke

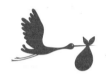

Always... be a little
kinder than necessary.

J. M. Barrie

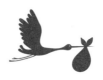

It goes without saying
that you should never have
more children than you
have car windows.

Erma Bombeck

There is no velvet so soft as a mother's lap, no rose as lovely as her smile.

Edward Thompson

Being a dad is
more important
than football.

David Beckham

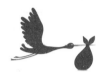

Never raise your hand
to your kids. It leaves your
groin unprotected.

Red Buttons

Biology is the least of
what makes someone
a mother.

Oprah Winfrey

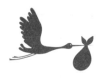

A baby is sunshine and
moonbeams and more,
brightening your world as
never before.

Anonymous

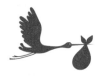

Think of stretch
marks as pregnancy
service stripes.

Joyce Armor

The quickest way for a
parent to get a child's
attention is to sit down and
look comfortable.

Lane Olinghouse

I think my life
began with waking
up and loving my
mother's face.

George Eliot

It's extraordinary to look
into a baby's face and
see a piece of your flesh
and your spirit.

Liam Neeson

The family you come from isn't as important as the family you're going to have.

Ring Lardner

You never understand
life until it grows
inside you.

Anonymous

A good father is one of the most unsung, unpraised, unnoticed, and yet one of the most valuable assets in our society.

Billy Graham

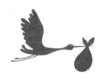

When you have
brought up kids, there
are memories you
store directly in your
tear ducts.

Robert Brault

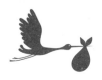

Making a decision to have
a child – it's momentous.
It is to decide forever to
have your heart go walking
around outside your body.

Elizabeth Stone

I've learned more from my daughter than she has learned from me.

Antonio Banderas

The mother's
heart is the child's
schoolroom.

Henry Ward Beecher

Do all things with love.

Og Mandino

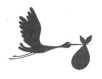

A father is someone who
carries pictures in his
wallet where his money
used to be.

Anonymous

It is not flesh and blood but the heart which makes us fathers and sons.

Friedrich Schiller

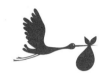

Always kiss your children goodnight, even if they're already asleep.

H. Jackson Brown Jr

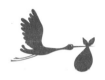

It is the most powerful
creation to have life growing
inside of you. There is
no bigger gift.

Beyoncé Knowles-Carter

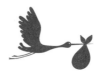

A mother's arms are
made of tenderness,
and children sleep
soundly in them.

Victor Hugo

I'm not going to have a
better day, a more magical
moment, than the first time I
heard my daughter giggle.

Sean Penn

Did you know babies
are nauseated by the
smell of a clean shirt?

Jeff Foxworthy

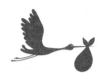

Family is not an important thing. It's everything.

Michael J. Fox

The toughest job in the
world isn't being a president.
It's being a parent.

Bill Clinton

There is no kind of affection
so purely angelic as of a
father to a daughter.

Joseph Addison

Our greatest natural resource is the minds of our children.

Walt Disney

Nothing beats
having this beautiful
child look at me
and say 'Mum'.

Nicole Appleton

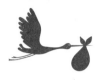

Don't ever tell the mother of
a newborn that her baby's
smile is just gas.

Anonymous

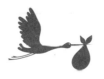

What is a home
without children?
Quiet.

Henny Youngman

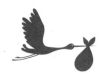

Getting a burp out of your little thing is probably the greatest satisfaction I've come across.

Brad Pitt

When you are dealing with a child, keep all your wits about you, and sit on the floor.

Austin O'Malley

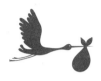

The gain is not the having of children; it is the discovery of love and how to be loving.

Polly Berrien Berends

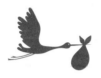

The moment a child is
born, the mother
is also born.

Rajneesh

A perfect example of
minority rule is a
baby in the house.

Anonymous

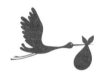

There's no road map on how to raise a family: it's always an enormous negotiation.

Meryl Streep

A father is a banker
provided by nature.

French proverb

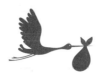

Children see magic
because they look for it.

Christopher Moore

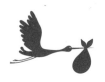

Being a mother
has made my life
complete.

Darcey Bussell

The worst feature
of a new baby is its
mother's singing.

Kin Hubbard

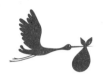

If you want your children to
listen, try talking softly –
to someone else.

Ann Landers

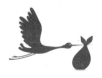

Parents who are afraid to
put their foot down usually
have children who step
on their toes.

Chinese proverb

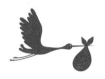

Sometimes
the strength of
motherhood is
greater than
natural laws.

Barbara Kingsolver

You have a lifetime to work, but children are only young once.

Polish proverb

The child supplies the
power, but the parents have
to do the steering.

Dr Benjamin Spock

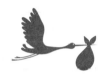

If your children look
up to you, you've
made a success of
life's biggest job.

Anonymous

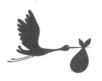

I studied pregnancy symptoms – moody, big bosoms, irritable. I've obviously been pregnant for twenty years.

Victoria Wood

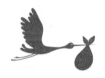

Childbirth classes neglect to teach one critical skill: how to breathe, count and swear all at the same time.

Linda Fiterman

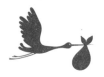

All babies are
supposed to look like
me – at both ends.

Winston Churchill

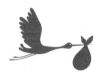

When my kids become wild
and unruly, I use a nice,
safe playpen. When they're
finished, I climb out.

Erma Bombeck

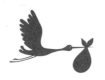

Being a dad is the new black.

Laurence Llewelyn-Bowen

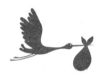

Even when freshly washed
and relieved of all obvious
confections, children
tend to be sticky.

Fran Lebowitz

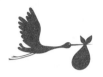

Wrinkles are
hereditary – parents
get them from their
children.

Doris Day

Children are like wet cement. Whatever falls on them makes an impression.

Haim Ginott

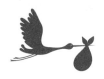

Of all the rights of
women, the greatest
is to be a mother.

Lin Yutang

Raising kids is part joy and
part guerrilla warfare.

Ed Asner

Children make your
life important.

Erma Bombeck

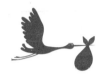

Everything comes
gradually and at its
appointed hour.

Ovid

This moment of meeting
seemed to be a birth time
for both of us; her first and
my second life.

Laurie Lee

Each day of our lives
we make deposits in
the memory banks
of our children.

Charles R. Swindoll

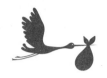

The fundamental job
of a toddler is to rule
the universe.

Lawrence Kutner

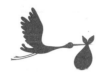

I love to think that the
day you're born, you're
given the world as your
birthday present.

Leo Buscaglia

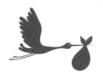

Pregnancy is a process that invites you to surrender to the unseen force behind all life.

Judy Ford

Children are a great
comfort in your old
age – and they help you
reach it faster, too.

Anonymous

Any mother could perform the jobs of several air traffic controllers with ease.

Lisa Alther

Human beings are the
only creatures on earth that
allow their children to
come back home.

Bill Cosby

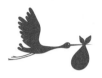

Never underestimate
a child's ability to get
into more trouble.

Stephen Wright

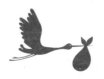

A baby is something you carry inside you for nine months, in your arms for three years and in your heart till the day you die.

Mary Mason

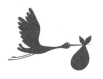

There are only two lasting bequests we can hope to give our children. One is roots. The other is wings.

Hodding Carter

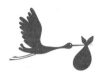

A child, like your stomach,
doesn't need all you can
afford to give it.

Frank A. Clark

There's no pillow quite
so soft as a father's
strong shoulder.

Richard L. Evans

Setting a good example
for your children takes all
the fun out of middle age.

William Feather

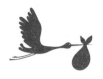

My mother had a
great deal of trouble
with me, but I think
she enjoyed it.

Mark Twain

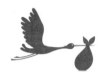

Parenthood: that
state of being better
chaperoned than you
were before marriage.

Marcelene Cox

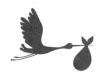

Children reinvent
your world for you.

Susan Sarandon

A sweater is a
garment worn by
a child when the
mother feels chilly.

Barbara Johnson

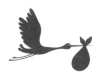

Aside from new babies, new mothers must be the most beautiful creatures on earth.

Terri Guillemets

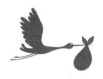

Families are like
fudge – mostly sweet
with a few nuts.

Anonymous

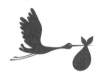

Before I got married I had
six theories about bringing
up children; now I have six
children and no theories.

John Wilmot

There was never a child so
lovely, but his mother was
glad to get him to sleep.

Ralph Waldo Emerson

The soul is healed by
being with children.

Fyodor Dostoyevsky

If evolution really works,
how come mothers only
have two hands?

Milton Berle

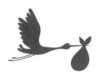

If the choice is
between sleeping and
the housework, sleep.

Anonymous

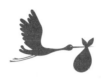

You can't understand it until you experience the simple joy of the first time your son points at a seagull and says 'duck'.

Russell Crowe on fatherhood

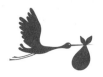

There is a power that
comes to women
when they give birth.

Sheryl Feldman

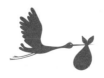

A child is not a
vase to be filled,
but a fire to be lit.

François Rabelais

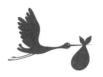

Babies are bits of
stardust blown from
the hand of God.

Larry Barretto

Having children gives
your life a purpose. Right
now, my purpose is to
get some sleep.

Reno Goodale

If men had to
have babies, they
would only ever
have one each.

Diana, Princess of Wales

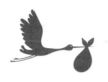

A mother always
has to think twice:
once for herself and
once for her child.

Sophia Loren

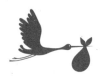

Birth is an experience that
demonstrates that life is not
merely function and utility,
but form and beauty.

Christopher Largen

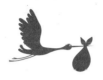

Anyone who thinks the art of conversation is dead ought to tell a child to go to bed.

Robert Gallagher

I'm not interested in being Wonder Woman in the delivery room. Give me drugs.

Madonna

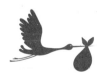

Loving a baby is a circular
business... the more you
give the more you get.

Penelope Leach

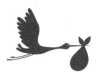

Kids spell love T-I-M-E.

Anonymous

To describe my
mother would be to write
about a hurricane in
its perfect power.

Maya Angelou

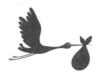

Your children need
your presence more
than your presents.

Jesse Jackson

Life doesn't come
with an instruction
book; that's why we
have fathers.

H. Jackson Brown Jr

The voice of parents is the voice of gods,
For to their children they are heaven's lieutenants.

William Shakespeare

Children must be
taught how to think,
not what to think.

Margaret Mead

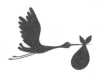

To witness the birth of a
child is our best opportunity
to experience the meaning
of the word 'miracle'.

Paul Carvel

Children use all their
wiles to get their way with
adults. Adults do the
same with children.

Mason Cooley

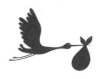

Insanity is hereditary
– you get it from
your kids.

Anonymous

A person soon learns
how little he knows
when a child begins to
ask questions.

Richard L. Evans

I understood once I held
a baby in my arms, why
some people have the need
to keep having them.

Spalding Gray

There was never a
great man who had not
a great mother.

Olive Schreiner

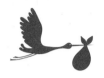

One father is more
than a hundred
schoolmasters.

George Herbert

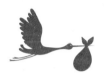

There is no reciprocity.
Men love women, women
love children. Children
love hamsters.

Alice Thomas Ellis

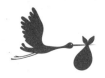

Every beetle is a
gazelle in the eyes of
its mother.

Moorish proverb

Parents learn a lot
from their children
about coping with life.

Muriel Spark

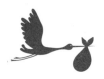

A man's children and his garden both reflect the amount of weeding done during the growing season.

Anonymous

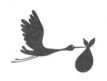

A grand adventure
is about to begin.

A. A. Milne

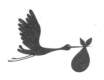

A home birth is preferable.
That way you're not missing
anything on television.

Jeremy Hardy

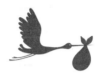

A two-year-old is kind of like having a blender, but you don't have a top for it.

Jerry Seinfeld

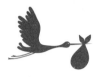

You can learn
many things from
children. How much
patience you have,
for instance.

Franklin P. Jones

A baby is born with a
need to be loved – and
never outgrows It.

Frank A. Clark

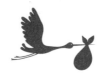

When they placed
you in my arms, you
slipped into my heart.

Anonymous

You will always
be your child's
favourite toy.

Vicki Lansky

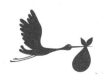

There is no way to be a perfect mother, and a million ways to be a good one.

Jill Churchill

Fatherhood is
pretending the present
you love most is soap
on-a-rope.

Bill Cosby

Having a baby is like falling in love again, both with your husband and your child.

Tina Brown

The hand that rocks the cradle is usually attached to someone who isn't getting enough sleep.

John Fiebig

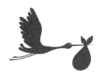

Every baby needs a lap.

Henry Robin

If you're interested in finding
out more about our books,
find us on Facebook at
Summersdale Publishers
and follow us on Twitter at
@Summersdale.

www.summersdale.com

KEEP CALM YOU'RE HAVING A BABY

KEEP
CALM
YOU'RE
HAVING A
BABY

KEEP
CALM
YOU'RE
HAVING A
BABY

KEEP
CALM
YOU'RE
HAVING A
BABY

KEEP
CALM
YOU'RE
HAVING A
BABY

KEEP
CALM
YOU'RE
HAVING A
BABY

KEEP
CALM
YOU'RE
HAVING A
BABY

KEEP
CALM
YOU'RE
HAVING A
BABY

KEEP
CALM
YOU'RE
HAVING A
BABY

KEEP
CALM
YOU'RE
HAVING A
BABY

KEEP
CALM
YOU'RE
HAVING A
BABY